Alkaline Transition Recipe Book

Discover a Revolutionary Way of Eating and Living to Support Dr. Sebi's Alkaline Way of Life

Isabelle Simonette

© Copyright 2024 by Isabelle Simonette - All rights reserved.
The content of this book may not be reproduced, duplicated, or transmitted without the direct written consent of the author or the publisher.

In no event shall the publisher, or the author, be liable for any fault or legal liability for any damages, repairs, or monetary losses due to the information contained in this book. Both directly and indirectly.

Disclaimer:

Please note, the following book is reproduced below with the goal of providing information that is as accurate and reliable as possible. Regardless, purchasing this Book can be seen as consent to the fact that both the publisher and the author of this book are in no way experts on the topics discussed within and that any recommendations or suggestions that are made herein are for entertainment purposes only. Professionals should be consulted as needed prior to undertaking any of the action endorsed herein. This declaration is deemed fair and valid by both the American Bar Association and the Committee of Publishers Association and is legally binding throughout the United States. Furthermore, the transmission, duplication, or reproduction of any of the following work including specific information will be considered an illegal act irrespective of if it is done electronically or in print. This extends to creating a secondary or tertiary copy of the work or a recorded copy and is only allowed with the express written consent from the Publisher. All additional right reserved. The information in the following pages is broadly considered a truthful and accurate account of facts and as such, any inattention, use, or misuse of the information in question by the reader will render any resulting actions solely under their purview. There are no scenarios in which the publisher or the original author of this work can be in any fashion deemed liable for any hardship or damages that may befall them after undertaking information described herein. Additionally, the information in the following pages is intended only for informational purposes and should thus be thought of as universal. As befitting its nature, it is presented without assurance regarding its prolonged validity or interim quality. Trademarks that are mentioned are done without written consent and can in no way be considered an endorsement from the trademark holder.

Table of Contacts

Chapter 1: Understanding The Alkaline Approach: What It Is and Why It Matters 9

    Achieving Health Through Balance: Acidic vs. Alkaline Cells .. 9

        The Impact of Diet: "Just a Burger and a Cup of Coffee..." ..10

        Maintaining Balance: The Importance of pH Levels............10

        Guarding Against Diabetes 11

        Supporting Kidney Health 11

        Strengthening Bones 11

Chapter 2: The Seven Principles of Alkaline Eating 13

    Eat a Wide Range of Fresh, High-Quality Whole Foods.......... 14

    Incorporate 60-80% Alkaline-Forming Foods 14

    Choose Immune-Friendly Foods.. 15

    Balance Your Intake 15

    Incorporate Probiotic and Fermented Foods and Drinks........ 18

    Ensure Ample Fiber and Water Intake 19

    Combine Foods for Better Digestion and Health 20

Chapter 3: Alkaline Recipes and Menus 23

    Breakfast Options... 24

        Alkaline Quinoa Breakfast Bowl (Serves 4)......................... 24

        Nutty Steel-Cut Oats (Serves 4).. 25

    Millet Berry Porridge (Serves 4) 26

    Rice Breakfast Porridge (Serves 4 to 6) 27

    Sunchoke Breakfast Hash (Serves 4) 28

Salads 29

    Sweet Garden Salad with Mint Dressing (Serves 4-6) 29

    Spring Greens and Apple Salad (Serves 4-6) 30

    Clementine Kale Salad (Serves 4-6) 31

Dressings, Dips, and Beverages 32

    Almond Green Goddess Dressing.. 32

    Sunflower Seed Dressing 33

    Dill Tahini Dressing.. 34

    Cashew Honey Dip.. 35

    Curried Pumpkin Dip 35

    Making Ghee... 36

Nut Milk Recipes 37

    Almond-Coconut Milk 37

    Almond-Cashew Milk 38

    Coconut Milk 39

    Fruit and Wine Spritzers 40

Lunch and Dinner Ideas.. 40

    Indian Lentil Dal (Serves 4-6) 40

    Vegetable Chili (Serves 4-6) 42

Vegetable Yum Soup (Serves 4-6) 43
Nutritious Desserts 44
Raw Chocolate Pudding (Serves 4)..................................... 44
Decadent Figs (Serves 4) 45

Chapter 4: Substitute Reactives..47
Be Nice to Your Immune System..47
Replacing Reactive Foods 48
Wheat Alternatives 48
Gluten Alternatives 51
Corn Alternatives... 52
Corn-free Meals 53
Cow Dairy Alternatives 54
Dairy-free Meals 56
Yeast Alternatives 58
Egg Alternatives... 60
Sugar Alternatives 62
Soy Alternatives 63
Avoiding Industrialized Animal Products 64
Sulfite Alternatives 65
Trans Fats and Hydrogenated Oil Alternatives 65

Chapter 5: Detox and Cleanse Guides...67
Essentials of Cleansing and Detoxification 67

Effective Detoxification Techniques 68

Liquid-Only Days 69

Benefits of Salt and Soda Baths... 70

The Role of Low-Temperature Saunas................................. 71

Additional Detoxification Techniques.................................. 71

Enhancing Detox with Healthy Habits 72

Chapter 6: Practices for a Healthy Mind and Body 75

Walking and Low-Impact Aerobic Exercises 76

Breath Work: Harnessing the Power of Conscious Breathing . 81

Chapter 7: The Role of Sleep in Health and Well-being 85

Chapter 8: Alkalinization and Health: Insights from Dr. Sebi ... 93

The Alkaline Diet... 94

Benefits of Alkalinization 99

Alkalinization and Disease... 100

Dr. Sebi's Herbal Remedies...102

Practical Tips for Transitioning to an Alkaline Lifestyle........104

Recipes and Meal Plans...106

Testimonials and Success Stories.. 108

Embracing the Alkaline Lifestyle for Optimal Health............ 110

Appendix A: Testing Your First Morning Urine pH 115

Appendix B: Transit Time Digestion Evaluation................ 117

Chapter 1: Understanding The Alkaline Approach: What It Is and Why It Matters

The Alkaline Approach is founded on over forty years of global research focused on enhancing quality of life and maintaining health and happiness.

Since we are the result of what we eat, drink, think, and do, it's essential to remember that optimal health and happiness depend more on choice than chance. This guide is designed to inform you, so you can make healthier choices for your body, mind, and spirit. It provides everything needed to support your body's natural immune defense, repair systems, digestion, detoxification, and neurohormone functions. The goal is to prevent illness by fully and safely meeting your body's needs. Moreover, following the Alkaline Approach in diet and mindfulness can inspire, motivate, and create a profound sense of well-being and resilience.

Achieving Health Through Balance: Acidic vs. Alkaline Cells

Health is all about balance. Our cells constantly strive to maintain an alkaline state. Even a slight shift toward acidity is linked to increased disease and reduced cellular resilience. When our bodies are more acidic, they become weaker and more susceptible to illness. Conversely, in a more alkaline state, our bodies are stronger and more capable of resisting and recovering from illness.

Our food choices significantly impact our health by affecting our acid-alkaline balance. Measuring our pH, as detailed in Appendix A: Testing Your Acid-Alkaline Balance, shows whether our bodies are in a healthy state.

The Impact of Diet: "Just a Burger and a Cup of Coffee..."

A diet high in fat, processed foods, sugar, and protein—common in the American diet—makes our bodies more acidic and less resilient, a state called metabolic acidosis. On the other hand, a diet rich in greens, plants, fruits, vegetables, minerals, and antioxidants makes our cells more alkaline and resistant to stress. Even a slight change in diet can dramatically impact our health.

Maintaining Balance: The Importance of pH Levels

Our pH level measures how acidic or alkaline we are, with 0 being completely acidic, 14 completely alkaline, and 7 neutral. Our bodies strive to maintain a slightly alkaline pH of around 7.35 in the blood. The foods we eat affect our pH balance, impacting our overall health. The typical American diet (meat, dairy, eggs, sugar, soda, coffee, tea, alcohol, nicotine, processed foods) is often imbalanced, increasing our acid load and risk of health issues.

An excess acid load burdens our bodies, making it harder to resist sickness and recover from stress, leading to fatigue, illness, and higher infection risks. In contrast, a balanced, more alkaline body pH can lead to less illness, lower cancer risk, better digestion, more energy, restful sleep, reduced yeast and parasite issues, increased mental alertness, and more.

Guarding Against Diabetes

Studies indicate that even slight metabolic acidosis can cause insulin resistance and hypertension. An acidic diet, combined with excess weight, lack of exercise, and aging, may result in metabolic syndrome and type 2 diabetes, which can impair cardiovascular health. Conversely, increased intake of fruits and vegetables and healthy lifestyle practices, as outlined in The Alkaline Approach, are linked to lower risks of diabetes and cardiovascular conditions.

Supporting Kidney Health

An alkaline diet supports and protects kidney health—one of our most vital organ systems. The kidneys remove waste, control blood pressure, and keep bones healthy. An alkaline diet can reduce the risk of kidney disorders, such as kidney stones, disease, and failure.

Strengthening Bones

Over 40 million Americans suffer from bone loss (osteoporosis or osteopenia), a major cause of hip fractures. Research now widely accepts that an acidic diet plays a key role in bone loss by increasing mineral loss from bones and joints, where minerals like magnesium and calcium are stored.

The Alkaline Approach is a holistic approach combining diet/nutrition and lifestyle practices to restore essential balance to the body. Recognizing that we are shaped by what we eat, drink, think, and do, the Alkaline Approach philosophy promotes balance through:

- Healthy nutrition that promotes alkalinity
- Avoiding foods that cause immune intolerance
- Staying well-hydrated
- Using supplements wisely
- Engaging in gentle detox practices
- Practicing low-impact exercise
- Adopting mind-body wellness approaches

Chapter 2: The Seven Principles of Alkaline Eating

Guidelines for Eating:

1. Diverse, fresh, high-quality whole foods

2. 60% alkaline foods for maintenance; 80% for recovery

3. Foods that support your immune system

4. 60-70% plant-based complex carbs; 15-20% protein; 15-20% healthy fats

5. Probiotic and fermented foods and drinks

6. Ample fiber and water

7. Tasty and healthier food combinations

Eat a Wide Range of Fresh, High-Quality Whole Foods

The foundation of the Alkaline Approach is primarily consuming whole foods, preferably organically or biodynamically grown. Emphasize plant-based foods like fresh vegetables and fruits, lightly toasted nuts and seeds, lightly steamed vegetables, sprouted grains and beans, fermented foods, and freshly squeezed juices. These foods retain active enzymes that promote digestion.

For maximum health benefits, include a variety of whole foods in your diet. Repeatedly eating the same foods can limit digestive and nutritional diversity and increase the risk of food sensitivities if digestion is compromised. Experiment with new flavors to enhance your palate and health.

Incorporate 60-80% Alkaline-Forming Foods

The second principle focuses on selecting predominantly alkaline foods. For those in good health, aim to consume at least 60% alkaline-forming foods. If you have a compromised immune system or need health recovery, increase to 80% alkaline-forming foods to help calm your immune system and support digestion.

Choose Immune-Friendly Foods

Once you have your list of reactive foods, eliminate them from your diet. Chapter 4: Substituting for Reactive Foods offers many healthy and delicious alternatives for common allergens.

Many people find that switching to non-reactive foods and following the Alkaline Approach leads to effortless weight loss and improved metabolism. Likewise, those who are underweight often gain healthy weight due to enhanced protein synthesis and repair from a health-promoting diet.

Balance Your Intake

60-70% Plant-Based Complex Carbs, 15-20% Protein, 15-20% Healthy Fats

Our fourth Alkaline Approach principle emphasizes maintaining a healthy ratio of complex carbohydrates, proteins, and fats.

Recommended Ratios:

- 60–70% of calories from whole food (plant-based) complex carbohydrates
- 15–20% of calories from protein
- 15–20% of calories from healthy fats (including plenty of omega-3 fats)

Whole Food (Plant-based) Complex Carbohydrates:

Unless otherwise directed by your healthcare practitioner, your Alkaline Approach eating plan should be rich in complex carbohydrates from vegetables, whole grains, legumes (beans, peas, lentils), and include seasonings, spices, and herbs. These should make up about 60-70% of your food intake.

Quality Protein:

Proteins should account for approximately 15-20% of your total calorie intake. About 50 to 60 grams of protein per day is sufficient for most people. Protein sources may include organic eggs and dairy products, whey protein, and deep cold-water fish like mackerel, sardines, tuna, herring, and salmon. Additional sources include nuts and seeds, sprouts, nutritional yeast, blue-green algae, miso, and mushrooms. You can also create "complementary proteins" by pairing grains with beans or dairy. Protein requirements may be higher if you are pregnant, recovering from illness, exercising intensively, or have other specific needs. Consult with your healthcare practitioner if you have special circumstances.

Healthy Fats:

Fat should constitute 15-20% of your daily calories. Focus on healthy omega-3 essential fats, which enhance energy production, protein synthesis, and tissue repair. Food-based sources of protective omega-3 fats include fresh nuts and seeds, cold-pressed organic oils like avocado, olive, safflower, flaxseed, walnut, sesame, peanut, and deep-sea fish oils. Other sources include borage, black currant, grape-seed, evening primrose oils, and Udo's oil™. Unless you consume oily, deep-water fish more than three times per week, omega-3 supplements are recommended. Ensure omega-3 supplements are sourced from uncontaminated sources and processed without oxidation.

Avoid Trans Fats and Hydrogenated Oils:

Trans fatty acids are harmful and handled by the body like natural saturated fats but with negative effects. They can cross the placenta, are stored in fetal tissue, and cause long-term cellular issues. Unfortunately, trans fats are common in fried foods, processed foods, and many conventional cooking oils, bakery goods, and candies.

Use unsaturated, non-hydrogenated, expeller-pressed, and preferably organic oils like olive, grapeseed, coconut, and peanut, along with exotic oils like avocado, almond, and mustard seed. Avoid solid cooking fats such as margarine, hydrogenated vegetable oils, lard, and Crisco, as well as deep-fried fast food. Hydrogenated oils can interfere with liver enzymes, raise cholesterol levels, negatively affect immune function, and promote certain tumors.

Incorporate Probiotic and Fermented Foods and Drinks

The fifth principle of The Alkaline Approach encourages regularly consuming a variety of probiotic (cultured or fermented) foods and drinks. Probiotics promote life by supporting a healthy gastrointestinal tract filled with beneficial bacteria that keep our bodies and immune systems balanced. Poor diet, stress, illness, and antibiotics can deplete these beneficial bacteria, allowing pathogens to thrive. Consuming probiotics helps colonize the gut with these beneficial bacteria.

Some Probiotic-rich Foods and Drinks:

- Kombucha (fermented tea)
- Kefir (fermented milk)
- Yogurt (dairy or nondairy, with live cultures)
- Sauerkraut (fermented cabbage)
- Kimchi (spicy fermented cabbage)
- Tempeh (fermented soybeans)
- Microalgae (freeze-dried)
- Hatcho Miso soup
- Pickles
- Olives
- Natto (fermented soybean)

Ensure Ample Fiber and Water Intake

The sixth principle of The Alkaline Approach emphasizes the importance of consuming sufficient fiber and water. Most Americans consume far too little of both. Traditional cultures free of Western degenerative diseases typically consume 40-100 grams of dietary fiber daily from whole, vibrant foods, while Americans average only about 10 grams.

Aim for at least 40 grams of fiber daily. Fiber adds bulk and softness to stools, promoting a healthy transit time from food consumption to waste elimination. Adequate fiber helps eliminate wastes easily and regularly, reducing the likelihood of toxic waste reabsorption into circulation. A healthy transit time ranges from 12–18 hours, minimizing the chance for unhealthy bacteria and yeast to thrive.

The Importance of Water:

Water intake is crucial, especially when consuming a high-fiber diet. Water aids fiber in efficiently moving wastes through the body, and every bodily system relies on water to function. Follow The Alkaline Approach by drinking at least one 8-ounce glass of purified water 8 times daily. For every 5-8 ounces of caffeinated beverages, add a glass of water. Avoid drinking water 20-30 minutes before and after meals to aid digestion. If you must drink during these times, limit it to small amounts of room temperature or hot water (or healthy tea), as cold water can slow digestion.

Fresh lemon juice, lime juice, or ginger can enhance the taste of water and act as digestive aids and alkaline enhancers.

Combine Foods for Better Digestion and Health

Smart food combining is an essential component of the Alkaline Approach. How we combine foods during meals can significantly impact digestion and overall health. The typical American meal—often a combination of meat (protein) and potatoes (starch)—is one of the least effective food combinations.

Healthy food combining is crucial for balanced nutrition and reduces digestive system stress. Pay extra attention to food combining if you experience digestive discomforts like acid reflux, bloating, leaky gut, heartburn, irritable bowel, or other digestive issues.

This guide provides basic principles of healthy food combining, but further reading and research are encouraged. The main principles are simplicity and compatibility. Here are some basic tips:

Food Pairing for Complete Proteins:

Plant proteins often lack some essential amino acids. Pairing foods based on their amino acid profiles can create complete proteins. For instance, brown rice and cooked beans lack certain amino acids when eaten alone but provide complete protein when combined.

Examples of Food Pairings for Complete Proteins:

- Beans and rice or corn
- Legumes with grains, nuts, seeds, or dairy
- Grains with dairy
- Dairy with nuts, seeds, and legumes

Simple Eating and Food Combining Tips for Optimal Digestion and Assimilation:

- Simple meals digest better.
- Do not overeat; eat until 75% full, leaving 25% for digestion.
- Eat faster-digesting foods first.
- Generally, consume fruit juice and healthy sweets alone (30 minutes before or 2 hours after a meal).
- Avoid combining concentrated proteins (meat, fish, eggs) with starches/carbs during weak or repairing digestion. Eat these at separate meals.
- Non-starchy vegetables pair well with everything except fruit.
- Avoid drinking cold water with meals, as it dilutes digestive juices. Drink warm water or broth to start any meal or 1 hour after meals.
- Lightly sip hot tea during or at the end of a meal to aid digestion.

Chapter 3: Alkaline Recipes and Menus

Our choices in eating, drinking, thinking, and actions shape our lives. These recipes are meant to inspire your creativity and provide nutritious ingredients to guide you. Adjust and season them to your taste, using the natural flavors of whole foods as your guide. Explore and experiment with both complementary and contrasting flavors for enhanced health benefits.

You can adapt almost any cuisine to an alkaline diet. There are numerous cookbooks, websites, and blogs with delicious and easy alkaline recipes. To help you get started, we've compiled some sample meals. These suggestions are nutritious and tasty, and you can customize them to your preferences (raw or cooked, sweet or spicy, etc.), making substitutions for any allergies or sensitivities.

Once you're comfortable with your new alkaline lifestyle, continue experimenting with a variety of alkaline-forming foods to create your own delicious recipes!

Breakfast Options

Alkaline Quinoa Breakfast Bowl (Serves 4)

Ingredients:

- 1 cup quinoa
- 2 cups water
- 1 cinnamon stick or ¾ tsp ground cinnamon
- 2-3 tbsp maple syrup

Toppings:

- ½ cup mixed berries
- 2 tbsp raisins
- 1 tsp lemon zest
- ¼ tsp grated nutmeg
- 3 tbsp whipped coconut cream
- 2 tbsp chopped nuts
- Optional: sheep or goat yogurt, maple syrup

Instructions:

1. Rinse quinoa thoroughly.
2. Combine quinoa and water in a pot, bring to a boil.
3. Add the cinnamon stick, cover, reduce heat, and simmer for 15 minutes.
4. Remove from heat, fluff with a fork, and mix in cinnamon and maple syrup to taste.

5. Add desired toppings and serve.

Macronutrient Estimates per Serving:

- Carbs: 30g
- Protein: 5g
- Fat: 4g

Nutty Steel-Cut Oats (Serves 4)

Ingredients:

- 3 ¾ cups water
- 1 ¼ cups steel-cut oats
- ¼ tsp salt

Add-ins:

- 1 tbsp almond butter or coconut milk
- 1 tsp cinnamon or ½ tsp nutmeg
- Mixed berries, diced mango, or dried fruit and nuts

Instructions:

1. Boil water, add oats and salt.
2. Reduce heat and simmer for 20–25 minutes, stirring occasionally.
3. Stir in almond butter or coconut milk for creaminess.

4. Mix in your choice of spices and fruits.
5. Serve warm.

Macronutrient Estimates per Serving:

- Carbs: 35g
- Protein: 6g
- Fat: 3g

Millet Berry Porridge (Serves 4)

Ingredients:

- 1 cup millet
- 2 cups water
- 1 cup milk of choice
- 1 ½ cups fresh or dried mixed berries
- 2 tbsp maple syrup
- ½ cup Greek yogurt or coconut cream
- 4 tbsp chopped nuts

Instructions:

1. Optionally soak millet overnight or toast for a nutty flavor.
2. Combine millet, water, and milk in a pot, bring to a boil.
3. Reduce heat and simmer for 15-20 minutes, stirring occasionally.

4. Top with cooked berries, yogurt or coconut cream, and nuts before serving.

Macronutrient Estimates per Serving:

- Carbs: 40g
- Protein: 6g
- Fat: 5g

Rice Breakfast Porridge (Serves 4 to 6)

Ingredients:

- 9 cups water
- 1 ½ cups short-grain brown rice or Haiga white rice
- ½ tsp salt

Toppings:

- Chopped hardboiled egg, scallions, cooked greens, shredded seaweed, brown sugar, toasted nuts and seeds, fresh or dried fruit

Instructions:

1. The night before, boil water, add rice and salt, cover, and let stand overnight.

2. In the morning, cook on medium-high heat, stirring until creamy.
3. Adjust consistency with water or soy milk as needed.
4. Serve with desired toppings.

Macronutrient Estimates per Serving:

- Carbs: 35g
- Protein: 4g
- Fat: 1g

Sunchoke Breakfast Hash (Serves 4)

Ingredients:

- 3-4 sunchokes, thinly sliced
- 5-6 Brussels sprouts, thinly sliced (optional)
- Sea salt and pepper to taste
- Drizzle of truffle oil or rosemary-infused olive oil (optional)
- Spring onion for garnish

Instructions:

1. After slicing, rinse sunchokes in cold water three times, then pat dry.
2. Warm a pan over medium heat, add oil or ghee, Brussels sprouts, and sunchokes.
3. Sauté until cooked through, about 4 minutes.

4. Garnish with spring onion before serving.

Macronutrient Estimates per Serving:

- Carbs: 15g
- Protein: 2g
- Fat: 4g

Salads

Sweet Garden Salad with Mint Dressing (Serves 4-6)

Ingredients:

- 2 cups garden sorrel leaves
- 1 head red leaf lettuce
- ¾ cup sliced nectarines
- 3 tbsp white wine vinegar
- 1 tbsp grapeseed oil
- 2 tbsp maple syrup
- ¾ tsp Dijon mustard
- 2 tbsp minced shallot
- 1 tbsp finely chopped mint
- 1 tbsp minced chives
- Salt and pepper to taste

Instructions:

1. Mix sorrel, lettuce, and nectarines in a large bowl.
2. Whisk vinegar, oil, maple syrup, mustard, shallot, mint, and chives in a small bowl.
3. Drizzle dressing over salad, toss lightly, and serve.

Macronutrient Estimates per Serving:

- Carbs: 15g
- Protein: 2g   Fat: 5g

Spring Greens and Apple Salad (Serves 4-6)

Ingredients:

- 8 cups mixed spring greens
- 1 celery heart, finely chopped
- 2 Granny Smith apples, thinly sliced
- 1 ½ tbsp olive oil
- Zest and juice of 1 lemon
- Salt and pepper to taste

Instructions:

1. Combine greens, celery, apple slices, and lemon zest in a bowl.
2. Drizzle with lemon juice and olive oil, season, and toss.
3. Serve immediately.

Macronutrient Estimates per Serving:

- Carbs: 10g
- Protein: 1g
- Fat: 7g

Clementine Kale Salad (Serves 4-6)

Ingredients:

- 2 cups kale, thinly sliced
- 1 ½ tbsp olive oil
- ¼ tsp salt
- 2 clementines, peeled and segmented
- 1 cup sliced baby carrots
- 3 tbsp clementine juice
- 1 tbsp lemon juice
- 1 tbsp raw honey
- Dash of vanilla extract
- Salt and pepper to taste

Instructions:

1. Massage kale with olive oil and salt until softened.
2. Add clementine segments and sliced carrots.
3. Mix clementine juice, lemon juice, honey, and vanilla, then drizzle over salad.

4. Toss and let sit for 5 minutes before serving.

Macronutrient Estimates per Serving:

- Carbs: 12g
- Protein: 2g
- Fat: 5g

Dressings, Dips, and Beverages

Almond Green Goddess Dressing

Ingredients:

- 1 cup almonds, soaked
- 2 cups water or vegetable stock
- Juice of 2 lemons
- ½ bunch chopped parsley
- 2 chopped scallions
- 2 cloves chopped garlic
- Sea salt or tamari to taste

Instructions:

1. Blend water or stock with lemon juice, parsley, scallions, garlic, and salt.
2. Gradually add almonds and blend until smooth.
3. Refrigerate before serving.

Macronutrient Estimates per Serving:

- Carbs: 4g
- Protein: 3g
- Fat: 7g

Sunflower Seed Dressing

Ingredients:

- 1 cup soaked sunflower seeds
- 1 cup water or vegetable stock
- Juice of 2 lemons
- ½ bunch chopped parsley
- 2 chopped scallions
- 2 cloves chopped garlic
- Sea salt or tamari to taste
- 2 tbsp fresh tarragon or ½ tsp dried thyme

Instructions:

1. Blend half the water or stock with lemon juice, parsley, scallions, garlic, salt, and tarragon or thyme.
2. Gradually add sunflower seeds and blend until smooth.
3. Adjust thickness with additional water if necessary.
4. Refrigerate before serving.

Macronutrient Estimates per Serving:

- Carbs: 5g
- Protein: 4g
- Fat: 9g

Dill Tahini Dressing

Ingredients:

- 1 cup tahini
- ⅓ cup fresh lemon juice
- 2 tbsp fresh or ½ tsp dried dill
- 1 tbsp garlic powder

Instructions:

1. Blend tahini and lemon juice.
2. Add dill and garlic powder, blending while adding water or stock to achieve desired consistency.
3. Refrigerate before serving.

Macronutrient Estimates per Serving:

- Carbs: 3g
- Protein: 4g
- Fat: 11g

Cashew Honey Dip

Ingredients:

- 1 cup raw cashews
- 1 tsp coconut oil
- 1 tbsp raw honey

Instructions:

1. Blend cashews, coconut oil, and honey in a food processor until smooth.
2. Adjust consistency with coconut water if needed.
3. Serve with sliced fruit.

Macronutrient Estimates per Serving:

- Carbs: 7g
- Protein: 3g
- Fat: 9g

Curried Pumpkin Dip

Ingredients:

- 2 cups grated pumpkin or butternut squash
- ½ sliced avocado
- 1 chopped tomato

- 1 sliced celery stalk
- 2 chopped scallions
- 2 tsp curry powder
- 2 tbsp lemon juice
- Sea salt or tamari to taste
- ½ cup water

Instructions:

1. Blend water and vegetables until smooth.
2. Add lemon juice, curry powder, and season with salt or tamari.
3. Adjust thickness with additional water if needed.
4. Refrigerate before serving.

Macronutrient Estimates per Serving:

- Carbs: 10g
- Protein: 2g
- Fat: 4g

Making Ghee

Ingredients:

- 1 pound (grade AA) unsalted butter

Instructions:

1. Melt the butter in a heavy saucepan over low heat.
2. Allow the butter to come to a slow boil, stirring occasionally.
3. Once a foam layer forms on the surface, reduce the heat and let it simmer for about an hour.
4. The butter will separate into three layers: foam on top, amber-colored clarified butter in the middle, and sediment at the bottom.
5. Skim off the foam using a fine-mesh skimmer.
6. Strain the clear ghee through cheesecloth into a clean jar.
7. Store in the refrigerator or freezer.

Macronutrient Estimates per Serving (1 tbsp):

- Carbs: 0g
- Protein: 0g
- Fat: 14g

Nut Milk Recipes

Almond-Coconut Milk

Ingredients:

- 1 cup raw almonds (soaked overnight)
- 1 quart water
- 1 cup shredded coconut

Instructions:

1. Blanch the almonds by pouring boiling water over them for one minute. Remove skins.
2. Blend soaked, blanched almonds with 1 cup of water until smooth.
3. Gradually add the remaining water and blend in shredded coconut.
4. Strain if desired.

Macronutrient Estimates per Serving (1 cup):

- Carbs: 2g
- Protein: 1g
- Fat: 4g

Almond-Cashew Milk

Ingredients:

- ½ cup raw almonds (soaked overnight)
- ½ cup raw cashews (soaked overnight)
- 1 quart water

Instructions:

1. Blend soaked almonds and cashews with 1 cup of water until smooth.

2. Gradually add the remaining water.
3. Strain if desired.

Macronutrient Estimates per Serving (1 cup):

- Carbs: 3g
- Protein: 2g
- Fat: 5g

Coconut Milk

Ingredients:

- 1 cup fresh coconut
- 1 cup water

Instructions:

1. Blend coconut with water until smooth.
2. Strain if desired.

Macronutrient Estimates per Serving (1 cup):

- Carbs: 6g
- Protein: 1g
- Fat: 8g

Fruit and Wine Spritzers

Instructions:

1. Fill a glass with fresh, ripe fruit (e.g., berries, pineapple, melon).
2. Add wine (optional) or fruit juice diluted with sparkling water.
3. Enjoy the crisp flavors and textures.

Macronutrient Estimates per Serving (without wine, 1 cup):

- Carbs: 15g
- Protein: 1g
- Fat: 0g

Lunch and Dinner Ideas

Indian Lentil Dal (Serves 4-6)

Ingredients:

- 1 cup red lentils (soaked)
- 2 green chilies
- ½ tsp cumin seed
- ½ tsp turmeric
- 1-inch piece ginger, grated
- 1 clove garlic, minced

- 1 medium onion, sliced
- 2 medium tomatoes
- 1 tbsp oil
- Salt to taste
- Chopped cilantro for garnish
- Juice of ½ lime (optional)

Instructions:

1. Soak lentils for at least 6 hours.
2. Boil lentils with turmeric until soft, then mash.
3. In another pan, heat oil and sauté onions, cumin, ginger, garlic, and turmeric.
4. Add chilies, tomatoes, and salt. Cook until well done.
5. Combine with lentils, bring to a boil, and add lime juice.
6. Garnish with cilantro and serve.

Macronutrient Estimates per Serving:

- Carbs: 20g
- Protein: 6g
- Fat: 4g

Vegetable Chili (Serves 4-6)

Ingredients:

- 2 tbsp vegetable oil
- 1 large onion, chopped
- 1 poblano chili, chopped
- 1 red bell pepper, chopped
- 3 cloves garlic, minced
- 2 jalapeño chilies, chopped
- 1 ½ tsp chili powder
- 1 ½ tsp cumin powder
- 2 cups cooked beans
- 2 ½ cup vegetable stock
- 3 tsp lime juice
- 4 tbsp chopped cilantro

Instructions:

1. Heat oil, sauté onions until translucent.
2. Add poblano chili, bell pepper, garlic, and jalapeño. Cook until tender.
3. Add spices, beans, and stock. Cook for 10-15 minutes.
4. Stir in lime juice and cilantro before serving.

Macronutrient Estimates per Serving:

- Carbs: 25g
- Protein: 7g   Fat: 5g

Vegetable Yum Soup (Serves 4-6)

Ingredients:

- 1 tbsp vegetable oil
- 1 garlic clove, minced
- 2 tbsp fresh ginger, grated
- 1 stalk lemongrass, minced
- ½ tsp crushed red pepper
- ¾ cup shiitake mushrooms, sliced
- 2 cups sweet potatoes, chopped
- ½ cup green bell pepper, chopped
- 5-6 cups vegetable stock
- 1 (14-oz) can coconut milk
- 2 tbsp low sodium soy sauce
- 3 tbsp chopped cilantro

Instructions:

1. Heat oil, sauté garlic, ginger, lemongrass, and crushed red pepper.
2. Add mushrooms, sweet potatoes, and bell pepper. Cook for 1-2 minutes.
3. Add stock, bring to a boil, reduce heat, and simmer for 10 minutes.
4. Add coconut milk and soy sauce. Stir and serve with cilantro.

Macronutrient Estimates per Serving:

- Carbs: 20g   Protein: 4g   Fat: 10g

Nutritious Desserts

Raw Chocolate Pudding (Serves 4)

Ingredients:

- 1 avocado, chopped
- 2 bananas, chopped
- 3 tbsp raw cacao powder
- 1 tbsp raw honey
- 1 tsp lemon juice
- 1 tsp coconut oil
- 2-3 tbsp coconut milk
- Unsweetened shredded coconut

Instructions:

1. Blend all ingredients until smooth.
2. Adjust with coconut milk for desired consistency.
3. Serve sprinkled with shredded coconut.

Macronutrient Estimates per Serving:

- Carbs: 20g   Protein: 2g   Fat: 10g

Decadent Figs (Serves 4)

Ingredients:

- 1 ½ lb fresh figs, quartered
- ½ cup Greek yogurt
- ¼ cup goat cheese
- ¼ cup ricotta
- ¼ tsp cinnamon
- 4 tbsp toasted walnuts, chopped
- 4 tbsp raw honey

Instructions:

1. Blend yogurt, goat cheese, ricotta, and cinnamon until smooth.
2. Spoon mixture into bowls, top with figs.
3. Drizzle with honey and sprinkle with walnuts before serving.

Macronutrient Estimates per Serving:

- Carbs: 25g
- Protein: 5g
- Fat: 8g

Chapter 4: Substitute Reactives

If you have known (immediate) or suspected allergies or intolerances, this section offers strategies for replacing common allergenic and difficult-to-digest foods. This approach can significantly ease the burden on your digestive and immune systems.

Be Nice to Your Immune System

A healthy immune system protects you from foreign invaders like viruses and bacteria and repairs your body after injuries. However, when your immune system is constantly defending you, it can't repair effectively. Over time, an overstressed immune system can become exhausted, increasing the risk of autoimmune disorders and chronic health conditions.

The main burdens on the immune system include remnants of incomplete digestion, food antigens, diabetes effects, and environmental allergens. By identifying and minimizing immune triggers, you can reduce the immune burden, allowing your body to return to a healthy and resilient state. This leads to improved, sustained health.

Replacing Reactive Foods

This section outlines steps to replace reactive foods with nonreactive alternatives. By avoiding inflammatory foods for three to six months (depending on the severity of your reactions), you allow your immune system to reset and restore. A well-functioning immune system is crucial for preventing chronic infections and diseases and recovering from any damage caused by inflammation. Once your immune system is highly functional, you can work towards lifelong health.

Wheat Alternatives

Wheat: Wheat is the most commonly used grain in the United States. Unless otherwise specified, "flours" usually refer to wheat flours.

Suggested Substitutions:

- Whole or ground grains: Wild rice, oats, barley, millet, quinoa, corn, couscous, amaranth, teff, buckwheat
- Starchy roots: Sweet potatoes, yams, turnips, parsnips, potatoes, yucca, Jerusalem artichokes
- Commercial wheat-free breads are available at food co-ops, health food stores, and specialty markets.

Wheat-free Eating: Wheat can be difficult to digest and is a common cause of allergic reactions. Read labels carefully to avoid wheat in breads, cereals, pastas, and crackers. Wheat may be listed under various names like durum, semolina, wheat germ, and more. Despite its prevalence, enjoyable wheat-free eating is possible with many alternatives available.

Basic Substitutions for Wheat:

- Nonreactive grains and root vegetables like baked potatoes, yams, parsnips, and winter squash
- Rice flour-based baking mixes and bread, rice cakes, and crackers
- Oriental rice noodles and bean noodles (ensure they are wheat-free)
- Sprouted breads and rolls
- Grain, flour, and pasta made from quinoa, millet, wild rice, barley, couscous, or Jerusalem artichoke
- Cooked cereals with steel-cut oats, buckwheat, corn grits, or millet
- Ready-to-eat cereals featuring organic puffed rice, corn flakes, puffed millet, amaranth, or 100% oat content
- Corn pasta and tortillas
- Spaghetti squash
- Commercial wheat-free breads and baking mixes

Contaminants and Grain Production: Grains are often contaminated with molds, insect parts, rodent hairs, and pesticides. Thoroughly wash all grains and use organic options to avoid contaminants.

Wheat-free Meals:

- **Breakfast:** Fresh vegetables and fruits, non-wheat cereals, pancakes, waffles, muffins made with wheat-free flours, eggs with wheat-free toast or almond butter on rice cakes
- **Lunch and Dinner:** Cooked vegetables with beans or meat, bean soups, stir-fried vegetables with meat or tofu, seafood with wheat-free pasta, broiled fish with root vegetables and salad, grain casseroles, wild rice with pecans, bean dishes, poultry soups, adapted comfort foods
- **Snacks:** Japanese rice balls, trail mix, wheat-free muffins or crackers, baked chips, fresh fruit, gelatin with fruit juice, fresh vegetables with bean dip, lettuce roll-ups, open-face sandwiches on rice cakes

Cooking and Baking with Wheat-free Flours: Non-wheat flours have unique textures and require more leavener like baking soda. Common substitutes include:

- 7/8 cup rice flour
- 5/8 cup potato flour
- 1 cup soy flour + ¼ cup potato flour
- 1 cup corn flour or finely ground cornmeal
- 1/3 cup soy flour, 1/3 cup potato flour, 1/3 cup rice flour
- ½ cup soy flour + ½ cup potato flour

Substitutes for Thickening:

- 1½ tsp cornstarch, potato flour, sweet rice flour, arrowroot starch, sago starch, gelatin
- 2 tsp quick-cooking tapioca flour
- 1 tbsp rice flour
- 1 tbsp kudzu per cup of liquid
- ½ tbsp (1½ tsp) agar agar per cup of liquid

Gluten Alternatives

Gluten: Gluten is a protein-rich substance found in wheat, rye, oats, spelt, Kamut™, and triticale. It is difficult to digest for many people.

Suggested Substitutions:

- Grains like millet, quinoa, wild rice, barley, buckwheat, amaranth
- Flours from beans, seeds, corn, potatoes, chestnuts, tapioca
- Root vegetables and tubers like sweet potatoes, yams, parsnips, turnips, winter squash, yucca, spaghetti squash, taro, Jerusalem artichokes

Gluten-free Eating:

- **Breakfast:** Polenta French toast, corn flakes, puffed rice, amaranth, corn grits, miso soup with vegetables

- **Lunch and Dinner:** Non-gluten grains with vegetables, bean soups, fish with vegetables, hummus with rice, corn tacos with refried beans
- **Snacks:** Baked sweet potatoes, fresh nuts and seeds, vegetables with bean dip, nut butters with gluten-free crackers, hummus with vegetables

Corn Alternatives

Corn: Corn is used in various forms like maize flour, corn sweetener, corn syrup, cornstarch, and corn oil. It is a common food allergen.

Suggested Substitutions:

- Grains like wheat, rice, barley, millet, quinoa, teff, potato starch, tapioca, triticale flours
- Sweeteners like honey, maple syrup, rice syrup, barley malt, Sucanat®, molasses, agave
- Cornstarch substitutes like kudzu, arrowroot, agar agar, gelatin, flours like taro or tapioca

Corn-free Eating:

- Avoid all forms of corn including corn syrup, mannitol, sorbitol, fructose, maltodextrin, and zein
- Read labels carefully to avoid corn components in commercial products

Basic Substitutions for Corn:

- Grains like wheat, rice, barley, millet
- Sweeteners like Sucanat®, molasses, maple syrup, stevia, raw honey, agave, date sugar, vegetable glycerin
- Cornstarch substitutes like arrowroot, kudzu, potato flour, agar agar
- High-carbohydrate vegetables like squash, sweet potatoes, yam, parsnips, yucca, turnips

Corn-free Meals

Corn-free Breakfast Ideas

- Fresh vegetable or fruit juice with yogurt.
- Non-corn cereals like cream of rice, oatmeal, rye, buckwheat, cream of barley, or amaranth.
- Corn-free baking mixes for pancakes, waffles, and muffins.
- Organic eggs or vegetable omelet.
- Puffed rice, millet, or wheat with dairy or dairy-substitute milks.

Corn-free Lunch and Dinner Ideas

- Seasonal steamed vegetables with fish, poultry (chicken, turkey, duck), or lamb.
- Vegetarian casseroles with tofu or beans and vegetables.
- Bean soups and stews.
- Stir-fried vegetables with meat or tofu.

- Avocado with rice and steamed vegetables.

Corn-free Snack Ideas

- Pretzels or baked potato chips.
- Rice crackers with nut butter.
- Fresh fruit.
- Sliced avocado with crackers.
- Vegetables with yogurt dip.

Corn-free Alcoholic Beverages

If you are reactive to corn or corn sugars, try tequila, 100% potato vodka, or Silverado 100% grape-seed vodka, avoiding corn-based alcohols, beer, and wine except for Cru and Grand Cru wines.

Cow Dairy Alternatives

Cow's Milk Dairy Products

These include butter, all types of cheese, and products made with cow's milk. Check labels for cow's milk proteins like casein, whey, lactoalbumin, and lactoglobulin, even in "dairy-free" foods.

Suggested Substitutions

- Milks made from rice, soy, oats, nuts (almonds, Brazil nuts, coconut, pine nuts).
- Goat's milk, goat/sheep cheeses, and yogurts.
- Fruit juice can substitute for milk in recipes.

- Blended banana and almonds or cooked potatoes for cow's milk.
- Soft tofu blended with water, lemon juice, and/or sea salt for soft cheese.

Dairy-free Eating

Avoid dairy products and hidden sources like Cool Whip, Coffee-mate, Irish Cream, and many nondairy creamers. Read labels to avoid dairy proteins.

Alternatives to Dairy in Baked Recipes and Soups

- Use water, fruit juice, or vegetable soup stock instead of milk or cream.
- Sautéed and pureed onions, carrots, or turnips can replace dairy in sauces.
- Coconut milk is great for creamed soups and Thai-style curries.

Alternatives to Cow's Milk

- Goat's milk, soy, rice, almond, coconut, hemp seed, and oat milk.
- Be cautious of dairy proteins in some nut or rice milks.

Alternatives to Butter

- Margarines, vegetable oil spreads, unrefined coconut oil, Earth Balance.
- Ghee, which can be casein, whey, and lactose-free (see Chapter 3 for a recipe).

Alternatives to Cheese

- Tofu can replace ricotta, cottage cheese, yogurt, or sour cream.
- Seasoned firm tofu for ricotta or cottage cheese.
- Blended soft tofu with water and lemon juice for yogurt or sour cream.
- Sheep or goat cheese based on tolerance.
- Nutritional yeast for a cheese-like flavor in cooking.

Dairy-free Meals

Breakfast Ideas

- Fresh vegetable or fruit juice, fresh fruit.
- Hot cereals like cream of rice, oatmeal, or barley with milk substitutes.
- Cold cereals with appropriate milk substitutes.
- Whole grain pancakes, waffles, or muffins with milk substitutes.
- Organic eggs or vegetable omelet with nondairy milk.

Lunch and Dinner Ideas

- Cooked low-carbohydrate vegetables with beans or fish, chicken, or turkey.
- Bean soups with cooked vegetables.
- Stir-fried vegetables with meat or tofu.
- Seafood with wheat-free pasta.
- Broiled or poached fish.
- Grain casseroles like Indian millet or wild rice with nuts or seeds.
- Bean dishes like twice-cooked beans in corn tortillas, red lentil dal, or vegetarian chili.
- Baked, roasted, or stir-fried chicken, or fresh chicken-vegetable soup.

Snack Ideas

- Fresh fruits.
- Fresh nuts and seeds.
- Rice crackers with hummus or almond butter.
- Soy milk or goat milk yogurt.
- Vegetables with dips made from eggplant, avocado, lemon juice, garlic, and herbs.

Yeast Alternatives

Yeast in Food

Yeast is used to flavor foods, leaven baked goods, and ferment foods. Avoid baker's and brewer's yeast, commonly found in breads, alcoholic beverages, vinegar, salad dressings, pickled foods, and many processed foods.

Suggested Substitutions

- Herbs and spices instead of yeast for flavoring.
- Baking soda, baking powder, or buffered vitamin C as leavening agents.
- Yeast-free crackers like rice cakes, matzo, rye crackers, corn tortillas, and popcorn cakes.
- Commercial yeast-free breads, sprouted-grain breads, macrobiotic breads, and unleavened chapattis.

Yeast-free Eating

Consume only unprocessed/unrefined foods while avoiding yeasts. Baker's yeast is used in all risen baked goods, and brewer's yeast is used in alcohol and vinegar production.

Alternatives to Baker's Yeast

- Baking soda and baking powder (preferably aluminum-free).
- Buffered vitamin C powder.

Alternatives to Brewer's Yeast

- Avoid alcoholic beverages and vinegars except for Bragg Organic Apple Cider Vinegar.

Yeast-free Breakfast Ideas

- Fresh vegetable or fruit juice with yogurt.
- Whole cooked grains like rice, corn, barley, rye, millet, amaranth, oats, or buckwheat.
- Cream of rice, rye, barley, or corn grits.
- Pure rice, millet, or wheat puffs; 100% oat cereal; corn flakes.
- Organic eggs or vegetable omelet.

Yeast-free Lunch and Dinner Ideas

- Cooked low-carbohydrate vegetables with beans, fish, chicken, turkey, or red meat.
- Bean soups with cooked vegetables.
- Stir-fried vegetables with meat or tofu.
- Seafood with whole grain pasta.
- Broiled or poached fish.
- Vegetarian chili or other bean dishes.
- Baked, roasted, or stir-fried chicken or fresh chicken-vegetable soup.

Yeast-free Snack Ideas

- Japanese rice balls with avocado or tuna.
- Trail mix with fresh nuts and seeds.
- Baked corn or potato chips.
- Fresh fruit.
- All-natural gelatin.
- Corn chips or potato chips with salsa.
- Hummus or baba ghanoush with vegetables or crackers.

Egg Alternatives

Eggs in Food

Eggs are versatile and nutritious, but alternatives are needed if you are sensitive to egg whites, egg yolks, or both. Duck and goose eggs rarely cross-react with chicken eggs.

Suggested Substitutions

- Arrowroot, ground flax, and fruit pectins like apricot or guava for egg yolks.
- Baking soda, baking powder, and buffered vitamin C powder for egg whites.

Egg-free Eating

Eggs are versatile, but nature provides many alternatives.

Substitutes for Egg Yolks

- Arrowroot powder for smooth texture, but thinner and less rich.
- Ground flax and fruit pectins for baking.
- Duck or goose eggs for those not allergic to them.

Substitutes for Egg Whites

- Reduce batter space to rise.
- Add lemon juice or vinegar to increase chemical activity.
- Triple the amount of baking soda or powder.

Egg-free Meals

Breakfast Ideas

- Fresh vegetable or fruit juice with yogurt.
- Whole cooked cereals like rice, corn, barley, rye, millet, oatmeal, buckwheat, quinoa, or amaranth.
- Cream of rice, rye, barley, or corn grits.
- Cold cereals like rice or millet puffs, 100% oat cereal, corn flakes, spelt flakes, flax, Kamut®, and kasha.

Lunch and Dinner Ideas

- Cooked low-carbohydrate vegetables with beans, fish, chicken, turkey, beef, or root vegetables.
- Bean soups with cooked vegetables.

- Stir-fried vegetables with meat or tofu.
- Seafood with pasta and vegetables.
- Broiled or poached fish.
- Grain casseroles like Indian millet or wild rice with nuts or seeds.
- Bean dishes like twice-cooked beans in corn tortillas, red lentil dal, or vegetarian chili.
- Baked, roasted, or stir-fried chicken or fresh chicken-vegetable soup.
- Egg-free sandwich with eggless mayonnaise.

Egg-free Snack Ideas

- Japanese rice balls with avocado or tuna.
- Trail mix with fresh nuts and seeds.
- Whole grain muffins or crackers (wheat-free are easier to digest).
- Baked corn or potato chips.
- Fresh fruit.
- All-natural gelatin sweetened with fruit juice.

Sugar Alternatives

Sugar in Food

Sugar is a common food additive, found in beverages, candy, ice cream, baked goods, peanut butter, alcoholic beverages, hams, juices, canned foods, vegetable dishes, frozen foods, salad bars, medications, lozenges, vitamins, and cosmetics.

Suggested Substitutions

- Honey, maple syrup, barley and rice malt, fruit juice concentrate, date sugar, fig concentrate, and carob.
- Evaporated whole cane juice.
- Stevia and agave as natural sweeteners.

Sugar-free Eating

Sugar addiction can lead to health issues like diabetes. Substitute with unprocessed honey, molasses, formaldehyde-free maple syrup, sweet spices, dried organic fruits, fresh fruit, and xylitol. Avoid artificial sweeteners like aspartame, Acesulfame K, and saccharine.

Soy Alternatives

Soy in Food

Soy is found in many forms like the bean itself, soy flour, soy oil, soy seasoning, soy protein, soy milk, tofu, miso, soy sauce, tempeh, and natto. Hidden sources include vitamin supplements, hydrolyzed vegetable protein, soy lecithin, soy isolate, and natural flavoring.

Suggested Substitutions

- Replace soybeans with different beans like kidney, black, pinto, white beans, chickpeas.

- Use sea salt, wine, mushroom broth, or other sauce preparations instead of soy sauce.
- Substitute soy protein with fish, fresh meats, beans, and a complementary protein like grains.
- Use almond, coconut, and other nut milks.

Soy-free Eating

Avoid soy in various forms and read labels carefully. Soy can interfere with hormones and is used widely in the food industry.

Basic Substitutions for Soy

- Fish, fresh meats, and beans with complementary grains.
- Whey protein bars and shakes.
- Replace soy sauce with sea salt, wine, mushroom broth, or other sauces.
- Use almond, coconut, and other nut milks.

Avoiding Industrialized Animal Products

Reducing animal products helps restore body chemistry balance. Factory-farmed meat poses hazards due to hormones, antibiotics, and unsanitary conditions.

Hazards of Supermarket Meat:

- Confined conditions, artificial lighting, conveyor belt feeding, and hormone-rich diets.

- Antibiotics induce pathogenic and antibiotic-resistant bacteria.
- Meat may be dyed for color and injected with chemical flavoring for taste.

Sulfite Alternatives

Read labels to avoid sulfites, which must be declared if over 10 parts per million (ppm) concentration.

Trans Fats and Hydrogenated Oil Alternatives

Trans Fats and Hydrogenated Oils:

Trans fats are linked to cardiovascular disease, high cholesterol, blood fats, and increased cancer risk. Hydrogenated oils interfere with essential fatty acid metabolism and are used in margarines, processed vegetable oils, mayonnaise, commercial peanut butter, baked goods, chocolate, and some carob products.

Suggested Substitutions

- Use non-hydrogenated "expeller-pressed", organic or biodynamic oils like olive, grapeseed, coconut, and peanut oils.

Chapter 5: Detox and Cleanse Guides

Understanding the Need for Detoxification

Detoxification is crucial for everyone aiming to enhance their health, maintain energy, and promote longevity. In today's world, our bodies are constantly exposed to environmental toxins that can disrupt metabolism and decrease efficiency. Detoxifying helps eliminate these harmful substances, facilitating recovery and healthier lifestyle habits.

Essentials of Cleansing and Detoxification

Initial Steps: Avoiding Harmful Substances

To embark on a successful detox journey, it is vital to avoid substances that place stress on your digestive and immune systems. These stressors are not only taxing on your body but also highly acidic, contributing to an imbalance in your body's pH levels.

Substances to Avoid During Detox:

- **Caffeine:** Found in coffee, black tea, cocoa, and colas.
- **Nicotine:** From all forms of tobacco.
- **Excessive Alcohol:** More than two ounces daily.

- **Nitrates:** Commonly found in deli meats and cheeses.
- **Certain Drugs:** Including amphetamines, barbiturates, narcotics, and PCP.
- **Pesticide Residues**
- **Solvents:** From recreational drugs, occupational, or hobby exposure.
- **Heavy Metals:** Such as lead, mercury, arsenic, cadmium, nickel, and aluminum.

Effective Detoxification Techniques

To detoxify effectively, consider integrating the following methods into your routine:

- **Resting the Digestive System**
- **Purification Techniques:** Such as low-temperature saunas and salt and soda baths.
- **Periodic Vitamin C Cleanse/Calibration**
- **30-Day Multisystem Detox Program**

Resting Your Digestive System:

In our busy lives, we often overeat and under-digest, placing a heavy burden on our bodies. Giving your digestive system a break can help alleviate this stress. Here are some methods to achieve this:

Liquid-Only Days

Designate one day each week (or part of a day) to consume only liquids. This practice allows your digestive system to rest without depriving your body of essential nutrients and calories.

Options for Liquid Days:

- **Vegetable Juice:** An excellent source of minerals, especially when made from organic vegetables. Carrot juice can be combined with other vegetables such as parsley, celery, spinach, cucumber, beets, and more. Adding ginger enhances digestion and alkalinity.
- **Vegetable Broth:** Made by simmering various vegetables, legumes, and beans. Season with sea salt, soy sauce, and herbs like oregano, basil, or thyme. Strain and drink the clear broth.
- **Miso Broth:** Preferably made with hatcho miso aged over 24 months. It's easy to digest and beneficial even for those with soy sensitivities.
- **Fruit Smoothies:** Blend ripe, tree-picked fruits into a puree for a delicious and nutritious drink.
- **Melon Juice:** Blend ripe watermelon or other melons. Add a bit of ginger tea to start the blending process.
- **Ginger Tea:** Made from fresh ginger root, steeped in hot water. It's refreshing at any temperature.
- **Lassi:** A traditional Indian drink made from active culture yogurt, blended with rose water and honey. Suitable for

those who can tolerate cow's milk, or use goat's milk or nut milk yogurt as alternatives.
- **Water and Citrus/Lemon Water:** Use deep spring water, naturally carbonated water, or water with citrus juice.
- **Herbal Teas:** Enjoy alone or with a squeeze of citrus juice or a touch of honey.

Benefits of Salt and Soda Baths

Salt and soda baths are an effective method to draw out fat-soluble toxins stored in your body. These baths help eliminate pesticides, PCBs, and solvents through the skin, improving mental and physical health.

Epsom Salt Baths:

- **Ingredients:** Half a cup of Epsom salts and half a cup of baking soda.
- **Instructions:** Dissolve in a tub of warm water. Soak for 10-15 minutes until your skin turns pink, not red.
- **Tips:** Massage your skin with a soft cloth. Add sesame oil for additional skin benefits, especially in cold weather. Shower afterward with a mild soap to rinse off the toxins.
- **Frequency:** Can be done daily.

The Role of Low-Temperature Saunas

Low-temperature saunas are another excellent way to detoxify. These saunas gently detoxify the body while providing a relaxing environment for the mind.

Sauna Methods:

- **Types:** Home sweat cabinets, home saunas, commercial saunas.
- **Temperature:** Lower (105–110°F).
- **Duration:** Longer (30–60 minutes).
- **Frequency:** 1–3 times daily, at least 3 times weekly, preferably 5 or more days a week.

After the sauna session, shower immediately using a mild soap to prevent reabsorption of the mobilized toxins. Use a loofah or gentle scrub brush for a thorough cleanse. A cool shower afterward can be invigorating and refreshing.

Additional Detoxification Techniques

Periodic Vitamin C Cleanse/Calibration:

A Vitamin C cleanse can help to calibrate your body's detoxification process. This involves taking a specific dose of Vitamin C to help flush out toxins. The process should be done periodically and under guidance to ensure it is effective and safe.

30-Day Multisystem Detox Program:

This comprehensive program involves a series of steps designed to detoxify multiple systems in your body. It includes dietary adjustments, supplements, and lifestyle changes aimed at enhancing your body's natural detoxification processes. This program should be followed for 30 days to achieve optimal results.

Enhancing Detox with Healthy Habits

In addition to these detoxification methods, adopting healthy habits can significantly enhance the detox process. Here are some recommendations:

Hydration:

- **Drink Plenty of Water:** Staying hydrated is crucial for flushing out toxins.
- **Herbal Teas and Infusions:** Herbal teas like chamomile, peppermint, and dandelion can support detoxification.

Dietary Adjustments:

- **Eat Organic:** Choose organic foods to minimize exposure to pesticides and other chemicals.
- **Increase Fiber Intake:** Fiber helps to bind and eliminate toxins through the digestive tract.

- **Incorporate Probiotics:** Probiotics support a healthy gut, which is essential for effective detoxification.

Physical Activity:

- **Regular Exercise:** Physical activity promotes circulation and sweating, which can help eliminate toxins.
- **Yoga and Stretching:** These activities can help reduce stress and support the body's natural detox processes.

Mental and Emotional Well-being:

- **Mindfulness and Meditation:** Practices like mindfulness and meditation can help reduce stress, which supports overall health and detoxification.
- **Adequate Sleep:** Ensuring you get enough restful sleep is vital for the body's repair and detox processes.

By incorporating these detoxification techniques and healthy habits, you can effectively support your body's natural ability to eliminate toxins. This comprehensive approach not only enhances your physical health but also promotes mental clarity and emotional well-being. Embrace the detox process as an opportunity to start fresh, rethink your health goals, and envision yourself in a healthier, more vibrant body.

Chapter 6: Practices for a Healthy Mind and Body

Integrating Healthy Habits for Mental and Physical Well-being.

While nutrition, supplementation, and regular detoxification are essential for maintaining an alkaline and healthy body, it is equally important to engage in practices that support mental and emotional health, as well as overall fitness. Both your mental state and physical activity levels significantly impact your body's acid load, long-term health, vitality, and resilience. This chapter explores various practices designed to reduce stress, promote mental clarity, and enhance physical vitality.

The Impact of Mental and Emotional Stress

Mental and emotional stress, along with physical inertia and tension, contribute to the accumulation of acid residue in the body. This residue depletes essential nutrients and hinders overall well-being. The following stress-busting lifestyle practices are designed to stabilize the mind, restore peace, and promote vitality.

Recommended Practices for a Balanced Life

To achieve and maintain a healthy mind and body, various practices can be helpful. These include walking, hatha yoga, Tai

Chi Chuan and Qigong, the Alexander Technique, the Feldenkrais Method, Pilates, and the Trager Method. Find a system that resonates with you and experiment until you discover what you enjoy and what benefits you the most. Regular practice over a sustained period leads to significant cumulative benefits.

The Importance of Conscious Movement and Breathing

Practices that combine movement with conscious breathing are highly recommended. Activities such as yoga and Tai Chi use breath to evoke a healing equilibrium. Alternating between gentle stretching exercises and more intense cardio or weight-bearing activities can be particularly beneficial, as the heart, a muscle, benefits from regular exercise.

Finding the Right Practitioner or Resources

Choose a practitioner you respect, someone who exemplifies the practices they teach. If a live instructor isn't an option, DVDs or books can be valuable supplements. The Resources section at the end of this chapter offers recommendations to help you get started.

Walking and Low-Impact Aerobic Exercises

Walking is an excellent form of exercise, whether it's brisk walking or a leisurely stroll. Aim to walk in a serene environment for at least 45 minutes every other day. Walking increases circulation and oxygen levels, and deep, slow breathing while walking accelerates lymph flow, a key detoxification system. Walking can also be integrated with mindfulness or meditation, further enhancing the body's natural healing abilities.

- **Pace Variations:** Start with slow, purposeful walking and gradually build up to brisk or speed walking.
- **Incremental Progress:** Begin with short walks and gradually increase the duration. For example, start with five minutes and add one minute each day.
- **Daily Integration:** Incorporate walking into your daily routine, such as parking further from your destination or choosing stairs over elevators.
- **Enjoyment and Motivation:** Link walking to activities you enjoy and track your progress with a journal or pedometer.

Physical Yoga – Hatha Yoga

Hatha yoga, a series of postures and positions developed in India, combines mindfulness and stretching. Yoga postures involve holding specific positions, moving rhythmically, and linking breath with movement. These practices enhance mindfulness, physical grace, stamina, and overall health. Yoga helps improve circulation, core strength, and organ function.

Yoga can be practiced with the guidance of a well-written book, video, or DVD. It's important to move at your own pace and not force your body. Find a style and teacher that resonate with you, and consider attending live classes to deepen your practice. Over time, yoga can enhance strength, serenity, energy, and flexibility.

Tai Chi Chuan and Qigong

Tai Chi and Qigong are ancient Chinese practices that enhance inner healing responses, oxygen delivery, immune function, detoxification, and brain function. These practices involve graceful movements and deep, relaxed breathing, creating a moving meditation.

To begin, find a book or video, and consider joining a class or practice group. Many hospitals, senior programs, and health centers offer Tai Chi and Qigong classes. Practicing with a mentor or partner can also be beneficial.

The Trager Approach

The Trager system, developed by physician Milton Trager, emphasizes the joy of natural movement. It helps release deep-seated tension patterns, promoting deep relaxation and a greater sense of aliveness. The practice can be done one-on-one with a practitioner or through self-induced movements known as Trager Mentastics.

Look for Trager practitioners or resources such as books and videos. Practice gentle, self-induced movements during daily activities to release tension patterns.

The Alexander Technique

The Alexander Technique focuses on realigning posture to decompress the spine, supporting deep breathing, elegant posture, and overall well-being. Developed by Mathias Alexander, this technique is effective for improving or resolving musculoskeletal conditions.

Find classes at community centers, hospitals, or through health plans. Books and videos can also guide you in practicing the Alexander Technique.

The Feldenkrais Method

The Feldenkrais Method, developed by Moshe Feldenkrais, helps individuals reconnect with their natural ability to move with awareness and grace. This method addresses dysfunctional habits of posture or movement, improving function and resolving pain.

Attend group classes such as "Awareness Through Movement" or individual lessons with a practitioner. Books and videos are also valuable resources.

Pilates

Pilates, developed by Joseph Pilates, focuses on core strength, spinal alignment, and improved coordination. This practice is used by a wide range of individuals, from dancers to athletes.

Practice Pilates mat work at home with videos or books, or join group classes at gyms, community centers, or studios. Advanced training on specialized equipment is also available.

Rebounder Trampoline

Rebounding on a mini-trampoline offers a unique, fun exercise experience. It provides aerobic exercise that reduces body fat and tones muscles, promoting a sense of youthfulness and relaxation.

Begin slowly and work up to at least 15 minutes twice a day. Instructional videos can help you get started.

Mindfulness Practices

Mental and emotional health is crucial for overall well-being. Mindfulness practices, such as meditation, help quiet the mind and create a sense of peace. These practices are especially important for those with chronic health conditions.

- **Choose a Practice:** Explore different forms of meditation, such as Vipassana or Zen, and find a teacher or resources that appeal to you.
- **Set a Routine:** Dedicate a specific time and place for daily practice. Create a meditation space at home or find a quiet place in nature.
- **Cultivate Non-Attachment:** Mindfulness meditation helps develop the ability to observe thoughts without reacting, promoting acceptance and discernment.
- **Consistency and Patience:** Practice daily for 20 minutes and consider intensive retreats. Remember, mastery takes time and dedication.

Breath Work: Harnessing the Power of Conscious Breathing

The healing traditions of every ancient culture have included some form of breath practice, reflecting the profound effect of the simple act of learning to breathe consciously. Deep breathing has the capacity to initiate healing and reduce the toll of stress on your body and psyche. Conscious breathing can:

- **Teach mindfulness:** Deep, deliberate breaths help anchor us in the present moment, promoting awareness.
- **Support energy levels:** Oxygen-rich blood energizes the body, improving overall vitality.
- **Promote relaxation:** Conscious breathing techniques can calm the nervous system, helping to maintain a relaxed state.
- **Serve as a refuge from stress:** Regular practice offers a reliable tool for managing stress and promoting emotional balance.

There are hundreds of breath practices to explore. To begin, we recommend incorporating deep, conscious breathing into your preferred movement-based practices. This combination can enhance the benefits of both activities.

Light Therapy: Illuminating the Path to Better Health

Photobiology, the study of light's interactions with living organisms, reveals how crucial light is for maintaining certain brain rhythms through daily fluctuations of light intensity and spectrum. Research links mood changes to these daily cycles, and studies suggest that appropriate lighting can alleviate seasonal depression (SAD).

To incorporate light therapy into your routine:

1. **Positioning:** Sit four to six feet from a Dichromatic Color green light for 20 minutes, twice a day—ideally in the morning and early evening. A socket-clamp light holder can help position the lamp effectively. You don't need to look directly at the light.
2. **Multitasking:** While receiving light therapy, you can perform other activities such as deep breathing, relaxation exercises, guided imagery, range of motion exercises, or reading. This can stimulate deep brain structures and chemical pathways.
3. **Multiple Lights:** Using several Dichromatic Color lights simultaneously can enhance the effects. Ensure these are the sole source of illumination in the room.
4. **Targeted Therapy:** If indicated by clinical experience, position amber/yellow or blue Dichromatic Color lights to shine on specific areas like the back, chest, or abdomen for

targeted benefits. The same duration and positioning conditions apply.

This light therapy approach builds on the early work of Edwin Babbitt, Dinsah Jadhiali, Faber Birren, Bhanté Dharmawara, and recent studies by Norm Rosenthal and Al Lewy.

Chapter 7: The Role of Sleep in Health and Well-being

While diet, exercise, and mindfulness practices are crucial components of a healthy lifestyle, sleep plays an equally vital role in maintaining overall health and well-being. Sleep is often overlooked in the pursuit of health, yet it is one of the foundational pillars of physical, mental, and emotional health. In this chapter, we will explore the importance of sleep, its impact on the body and mind, the consequences of sleep deprivation, and practical tips for improving sleep quality. By understanding and prioritizing sleep, you can enhance your overall quality of life and achieve a more balanced, vibrant state of health.

The Importance of Sleep

Sleep is essential for various physiological processes, including:

- **Physical Restoration:** During sleep, the body undergoes critical repair processes. Muscle tissue is rebuilt, and cells are regenerated. Growth hormone, which is vital for tissue growth and muscle repair, is primarily secreted during deep sleep. This restorative function is crucial for maintaining physical health and stamina.
- **Cognitive Function:** Sleep enhances memory consolidation, learning, problem-solving skills, and

creativity. The brain processes information acquired during the day, transferring it from short-term to long-term memory. REM (Rapid Eye Movement) sleep, in particular, is associated with improved cognitive functions and emotional regulation.

- **Emotional Regulation:** Adequate sleep helps regulate emotions, reducing stress and improving mood. Lack of sleep can lead to increased irritability, anxiety, and mood swings. It also impairs the ability to cope with stress and hinders emotional resilience.
- **Metabolic Health:** Sleep influences metabolism, appetite regulation, and weight management. Hormones that control hunger, such as ghrelin and leptin, are regulated during sleep. Poor sleep can lead to imbalances, increasing the risk of obesity, diabetes, and other metabolic disorders.
- **Immune Function:** Sleep strengthens the immune system. During sleep, the body produces cytokines, proteins that help fight infection, inflammation, and stress. Chronic sleep deprivation can weaken the immune response, making the body more susceptible to illnesses.

Understanding Sleep Cycles

Sleep consists of several cycles, each with distinct stages:

1. **Stage 1 (NREM):** Light sleep, where you drift in and out of sleep. This transitional phase lasts for several minutes as the body prepares for deeper sleep.
2. **Stage 2 (NREM):** Onset of sleep, where body temperature drops, heart rate slows, and brain activity decreases. This stage accounts for about 50% of the sleep cycle and is essential for processing memories and learning.
3. **Stage 3 (NREM):** Deep sleep, also known as slow-wave sleep, is crucial for physical restoration and immune function. During this stage, the body repairs and regenerates tissues, builds muscle and bone, and strengthens the immune system. It is harder to wake up during this stage.
4. **Stage 4 (REM):** Rapid Eye Movement sleep, characterized by increased brain activity, vivid dreams, and temporary muscle paralysis. This stage is crucial for cognitive function, emotional health, and memory consolidation. REM sleep occurs in cycles throughout the night, with each cycle becoming longer towards the morning.

Common Sleep Disorders

Several sleep disorders can affect sleep quality and overall health:

- **Insomnia:** Difficulty falling or staying asleep, leading to insufficient sleep. Insomnia can be caused by stress, anxiety, depression, poor sleep habits, or medical conditions.
- **Sleep Apnea:** Interrupted breathing during sleep, leading to frequent awakenings. This disorder can result in severe health issues, including cardiovascular disease and high blood pressure.
- **Restless Legs Syndrome (RLS):** Unpleasant sensations in the legs, causing an urge to move them, which can disrupt sleep.
- **Narcolepsy:** Excessive daytime sleepiness and sudden sleep attacks, often accompanied by cataplexy (sudden loss of muscle tone).
- **Circadian Rhythm Disorders:** Disruptions in the body's internal clock that regulate the sleep-wake cycle. These disorders can be caused by shift work, jet lag, or irregular sleep schedules.

Consequences of Sleep Deprivation

Chronic sleep deprivation can have severe consequences on health and well-being:

- **Cognitive Impairment:** Lack of sleep impairs attention, alertness, concentration, reasoning, and problem-solving. It also affects memory consolidation and learning.
- **Emotional Instability:** Sleep deprivation can lead to mood swings, irritability, anxiety, and depression. It also reduces the ability to cope with stress and increases emotional reactivity.
- **Physical Health Issues:** Chronic sleep deprivation is linked to a higher risk of cardiovascular diseases, obesity, diabetes, and weakened immune function. It can also lead to hormonal imbalances that affect metabolism and appetite regulation.
- **Accidents and Injuries:** Sleep deprivation increases the risk of accidents and injuries due to impaired judgment, slower reaction times, and decreased coordination. This is particularly concerning for activities that require full attention, such as driving.

Tips for Improving Sleep Quality

To enhance sleep quality, consider the following strategies:

- **Establish a Routine:** Go to bed and wake up at the same time every day, even on weekends. Consistency reinforces your body's sleep-wake cycle and can help you fall asleep and wake up more easily.
- **Create a Sleep-Friendly Environment:** Keep your bedroom dark, quiet, and cool. Use blackout curtains, earplugs, or white noise machines to minimize disturbances. Ensure your mattress and pillows are comfortable and supportive.
- **Limit Screen Time:** Avoid screens (phones, tablets, computers) at least an hour before bed, as the blue light can interfere with melatonin production. Instead, engage in relaxing activities like reading a book, taking a warm bath, or practicing relaxation exercises.
- **Mind Your Diet:** Avoid caffeine, alcohol, and large meals before bedtime. These substances can disrupt sleep by affecting your ability to fall and stay asleep. Opt for a light snack if you're hungry, such as a banana or a small bowl of oatmeal.
- **Exercise Regularly:** Engage in regular physical activity, but avoid vigorous exercise close to bedtime. Exercise can promote better sleep by reducing stress and anxiety, and improving sleep quality.

- **Practice Relaxation Techniques:** Try deep breathing, meditation, or gentle yoga to wind down before sleep. These practices can help calm the mind, reduce stress, and prepare the body for sleep.
- **Limit Naps:** If you need to nap, keep it short (20-30 minutes) and avoid napping late in the day. Long or late naps can interfere with nighttime sleep.

Natural Sleep Aids

If you're struggling with sleep, consider natural aids:

- **Herbal Teas:** Chamomile, valerian root, and lavender teas can promote relaxation and improve sleep. These herbs have mild sedative effects that can help ease anxiety and facilitate sleep.
- **Supplements:** Melatonin, magnesium, and tryptophan supplements may help regulate sleep patterns. Melatonin is a hormone that regulates the sleep-wake cycle, while magnesium and tryptophan play roles in muscle relaxation and serotonin production.
- **Essential Oils:** Aromatherapy with essential oils like lavender, cedarwood, or bergamot can create a calming atmosphere. These oils can be diffused in the bedroom or applied to the skin (diluted with a carrier oil) to promote relaxation and sleep.

Seeking Professional Help

If sleep problems persist despite trying these strategies, consult a healthcare professional. They can help diagnose and treat underlying sleep disorders or recommend further interventions. Cognitive-behavioral therapy for insomnia (CBT-I) is an effective treatment that can help change thoughts and behaviors that interfere with sleep.

Incorporating healthy sleep habits into your lifestyle is essential for maintaining physical health, cognitive function, and emotional well-being. By understanding the importance of sleep and implementing practical tips for improving sleep quality, you can achieve a more restful and rejuvenating sleep, ultimately enhancing your overall quality of life. Prioritizing sleep, along with diet, exercise, and mindfulness practices, can lead to a balanced, vibrant, and healthier you.

Chapter 8: Alkalinization and Health: Insights from Dr. Sebi

Dr. Sebi, born Alfredo Bowman, was a renowned Honduran herbalist who advocated for a unique approach to health centered around the concept of alkalinization. He believed that many diseases are caused by an acidic internal environment and mucus buildup resulting from consuming acidic foods. His philosophy emphasizes the importance of maintaining an alkaline internal environment to prevent and reverse disease, promote optimal health, and enhance overall vitality.

Dr. Sebi's approach is deeply rooted in African bio-mineral balance, a system that highlights the significance of natural, unprocessed foods. He was a vocal critic of Western medicine's approach, which often focuses on treating symptoms with pharmaceuticals rather than addressing the root causes of disease. Instead, Dr. Sebi proposed a diet rich in natural, plant-based foods that are "electric" – meaning they are alive and compatible with the body's natural electric composition. This holistic approach aims to restore the body's natural pH balance, support the immune system, and promote overall wellness.

Dr. Sebi's dietary recommendations are based on his extensive research and understanding of natural healing. He stressed the importance of avoiding foods that contribute to acidity and mucus buildup, advocating instead for a diet rich in alkaline-forming foods. His philosophy also includes the use of herbal remedies to cleanse and detoxify the body, enhancing its ability to heal itself naturally.

The Alkaline Diet

Dr. Sebi's alkaline diet is designed to support and maintain the body's natural alkaline state by emphasizing the consumption of natural, plant-based foods and avoiding processed and acidic foods. This diet is rich in minerals, vitamins, and nutrients essential for overall health, and it encourages the body to function optimally by maintaining a balanced pH level.

Key Principles of Dr. Sebi's Alkaline Diet:

- **Plant-Based Focus**: Dr. Sebi's diet is primarily plant-based, focusing on fruits, vegetables, nuts, seeds, and grains. This approach ensures that the body receives essential nutrients while avoiding the harmful effects of animal products and processed foods.
- **Natural and Unprocessed**: The diet emphasizes the importance of consuming natural, unprocessed foods. Processed foods often contain additives, preservatives, and artificial ingredients that can disrupt the body's pH balance and contribute to disease.

- **Electric Foods**: Dr. Sebi promoted the consumption of "electric" foods, which are natural and compatible with the body's electric composition. These foods are believed to enhance the body's natural energy and promote healing.
- **Hydration**: Proper hydration is crucial for maintaining an alkaline state. Dr. Sebi recommended drinking natural spring water and herbal teas to support the body's hydration needs.

Detailed List of Dr. Sebi's Approved Foods:

- **Vegetables**:
    - Amaranth greens
    - Avocados
    - Bell peppers
    - Burro bananas
    - Chayote
    - Cucumbers
    - Dandelion greens
    - Garbanzo beans
    - Kale
    - Lettuce (all types, except iceberg)
    - Mushrooms (all types, except shiitake)
    - Nopales
    - Okra
    - Olives
    - Onions
    - Squash

- Tomatoes (cherry and plum only)
- Tomatillo
- Turnip greens
- Watercress
- Zucchini
- **Fruits**:
    - Apples
    - Bananas (small or burro)
    - Berries (all varieties, except cranberries)
    - Cantaloupes
    - Cherries
    - Currants
    - Dates
    - Figs
    - Grapes (seeded)
    - Limes (key limes preferred with seeds)
    - Mangoes
    - Melons (seeded)
    - Oranges (Seville or sour preferred)
    - Papayas
    - Peaches
    - Pears
    - Plums
    - Prunes
    - Raisins (seeded)
    - Soft jelly coconuts
    - Soursops (Latin or West Indian markets)

- **Grains**:
    - Amaranth
    - Fonio
    - Kamut
    - Quinoa
    - Rye
    - Spelt
    - Teff
    - Wild rice
- **Nuts & Seeds**:
    - Hemp seed
    - Raw sesame seeds
    - Raw sesame tahini butter
    - Walnuts
    - Brazil nuts
- **Oils**:
    - Avocado oil
    - Coconut oil
    - Grapeseed oil
    - Hempseed oil
    - Olive oil
    - Sesame oil
- **Spices & Seasonings**:
    - Basil
    - Bay leaf
    - Cilantro
    - Coriander

- Dill
- Oregano
- Savory
- Sweet basil
- Tarragon
- Thyme

Foods to Avoid According to Dr. Sebi:

- **Animal Products**:
    - All meat
    - Dairy
    - Eggs
- **Processed Foods**:
    - White flour products
    - Artificial flavors
    - Colors
    - Preservatives
- **Stimulants**:
    - Coffee
    - Tea (non-herbal)
    - Alcohol
- **Hybrid and Genetically Modified Foods**:
    - Corn
    - Seedless fruits
    - Potatoes (except red and white)
    - Carrots
    - Beets

- o   Soy products
- o   Wheat

Benefits of Alkalinization

Dr. Sebi believed that maintaining an alkaline diet supports overall health and well-being by creating an environment in which disease cannot thrive. He asserted that an alkaline body is better equipped to resist disease and recover from illness. The benefits of adhering to an alkaline diet as proposed by Dr. Sebi include:

- **Disease Prevention**: An alkaline environment is less conducive to the development of chronic diseases such as cancer, diabetes, and heart disease. Dr. Sebi believed that by maintaining an alkaline state, the body can naturally ward off disease and support overall health.
- **Increased Vitality**: Consuming natural, plant-based foods provides essential nutrients that boost energy levels and enhance overall vitality. Alkaline foods are rich in vitamins, minerals, and antioxidants, which support the body's natural energy production and promote a sense of well-being.
- **Enhanced Digestion**: Alkaline foods support digestive health by reducing acidity and promoting a healthy gut environment. This can lead to improved nutrient absorption, better digestion, and a reduction in gastrointestinal issues such as bloating and indigestion.

- **Improved Mental Clarity**: A balanced diet that includes alkaline foods can improve cognitive function and mental clarity. Alkaline foods help reduce inflammation and oxidative stress in the brain, supporting better cognitive performance and mental health.
- **Weight Management**: Alkaline foods are typically lower in calories and higher in nutrients, which can support healthy weight management. By reducing the intake of processed and high-calorie foods, individuals can achieve and maintain a healthy weight.

Alkalinization and Disease

Dr. Sebi's approach emphasizes the direct relationship between body acidity and the development of disease. He argued that an acidic internal environment leads to mucus buildup, which in turn creates the conditions for disease to thrive. By maintaining an alkaline state, one can combat various illnesses and improve overall health.

Specific Health Benefits of an Alkaline Diet:

- **Cancer Prevention**: An alkaline environment is believed to inhibit the growth and spread of cancer cells. Dr. Sebi suggested that cancer cells thrive in acidic conditions, and by maintaining an alkaline environment, the growth of these cells can be slowed or prevented.

- **Diabetes Management**: Alkaline foods can help regulate blood sugar levels and improve insulin sensitivity. By reducing the intake of sugary and processed foods, individuals can better manage their blood sugar levels and reduce the risk of developing type 2 diabetes.
- **Heart Health**: Reducing acidity can lower the risk of cardiovascular diseases by decreasing inflammation and improving arterial health. Alkaline foods support the cardiovascular system by reducing plaque buildup in the arteries and promoting healthy blood flow.
- **Anti-Inflammatory Effects**: An alkaline diet can reduce inflammation throughout the body, alleviating symptoms of conditions like arthritis and asthma. By consuming foods that reduce acidity, individuals can lower inflammation levels and experience relief from chronic inflammatory conditions.
- **Detoxification**: Alkaline foods support the body's natural detoxification processes, helping to eliminate toxins and improve organ function. Foods such as leafy greens, fruits, and herbs aid the liver and kidneys in filtering and removing harmful substances from the body.

Dr. Sebi's Herbal Remedies

Dr. Sebi's philosophy on health and healing extends beyond diet to include a variety of herbal remedies. These natural plant-based solutions are designed to cleanse and detoxify the body, support immune function, and restore the body's natural balance. Dr. Sebi identified specific herbs that align with his alkaline principles and used them to create a range of products aimed at promoting health and reversing disease.

Key Herbs in Dr. Sebi's Regimen:

- **Burdock Root**: Known for its blood-purifying properties, burdock root helps detoxify the blood and lymphatic system. It is rich in antioxidants and supports liver function.
- **Sarsaparilla**: This herb is celebrated for its high iron content and ability to detoxify the blood. It also has anti-inflammatory and antimicrobial properties.
- **Elderberry**: Elderberry is used to boost the immune system, fight off colds and flu, and support respiratory health. It is high in vitamins A and C.
- **Bladderwrack**: A type of seaweed, bladderwrack is rich in iodine, which supports thyroid health. It also contains essential minerals that help detoxify the body.
- **Cascara Sagrada**: This herb is a natural laxative that promotes healthy digestion and bowel movements, helping to cleanse the colon.

- **Dandelion Root**: Dandelion root supports liver function and acts as a diuretic to help flush toxins from the body.
- **Chaparral**: Known for its powerful detoxifying effects, chaparral supports skin health and helps eliminate toxins from the body.

Dr. Sebi's Herbal Remedies for Specific Health Issues:

- **Immune Support**: A combination of elderberry, echinacea, and astragalus can boost the immune system, helping the body fend off infections.
- **Digestive Health**: Herbs like cascara sagrada, ginger, and peppermint can improve digestion, alleviate bloating, and promote regular bowel movements.
- **Detoxification**: A blend of burdock root, dandelion root, and sarsaparilla can cleanse the blood and liver, removing toxins and impurities.
- **Respiratory Health**: Mullein, licorice root, and elderberry are effective in supporting respiratory health and alleviating symptoms of colds and flu.
- **Skin Health**: Herbs such as chaparral and burdock root can help clear skin conditions by detoxifying the body and supporting liver function.

Practical Tips for Transitioning to an Alkaline Lifestyle

Transitioning to an alkaline lifestyle as advocated by Dr. Sebi requires gradual changes and a commitment to holistic health practices. Here are practical tips to help you make this transition smoothly and effectively:

1. Start Slowly: Begin by incorporating more alkaline foods into your diet gradually. Replace one meal a day with alkaline-rich foods, and slowly increase as you become more comfortable.

2. Educate Yourself: Read books, watch documentaries, and join online communities dedicated to Dr. Sebi's principles. Understanding the rationale behind the diet will motivate you to stick with it.

3. Meal Planning: Plan your meals ahead of time to ensure you have the necessary ingredients on hand. This can help prevent the temptation to revert to old eating habits.

4. Stay Hydrated: Drink plenty of spring water and herbal teas throughout the day. Staying hydrated helps maintain an alkaline state and supports overall health.

5. Prepare for Detox Symptoms: As your body adjusts to the new diet, you may experience detox symptoms such as headaches, fatigue, or digestive changes. These are normal and typically temporary.

6. Find Support: Seek support from friends, family, or online communities. Sharing your journey with others can provide encouragement and accountability.

7. Listen to Your Body: Pay attention to how your body responds to different foods and adjust accordingly. Everyone's body is unique, and what works for one person may not work for another.

8. Incorporate Herbal Supplements: Use Dr. Sebi's recommended herbal supplements to support your transition and enhance the detoxification process.

9. Practice Mindfulness: Incorporate practices such as meditation, yoga, or deep breathing exercises to support your mental and emotional health during the transition.

10. Be Patient: Transitioning to an alkaline lifestyle is a journey, not a quick fix. Be patient with yourself and celebrate your progress, no matter how small.

Recipes and Meal Plans

Embracing Dr. Sebi's alkaline diet can be both enjoyable and delicious. Below are some recipes and meal plans to help you get started on your journey to better health.

Breakfast Ideas:

- **Quinoa Porridge**: Cook quinoa with almond milk, add a touch of cinnamon, and top with fresh berries and a drizzle of agave syrup.
- **Smoothie Bowl**: Blend kale, spinach, banana, and mango with coconut water. Top with hemp seeds, sliced almonds, and fresh berries.
- **Amaranth Pancakes**: Make pancakes using amaranth flour, almond milk, and a dash of vanilla. Serve with pure maple syrup and fresh fruit.

Lunch Ideas:

- **Kale and Avocado Salad**: Massage kale with olive oil and lemon juice. Add avocado, cherry tomatoes, cucumber, and hemp seeds. Drizzle with tahini dressing.
- **Vegetable Stir-Fry**: Sauté zucchini, bell peppers, onions, and mushrooms in grapeseed oil. Season with tamari sauce and serve over wild rice.

- **Chickpea Wraps**: Fill a spelt tortilla with mashed chickpeas, diced tomatoes, cucumbers, and a drizzle of tahini sauce.

Dinner Ideas:

- **Stuffed Peppers**: Fill bell peppers with a mixture of quinoa, black beans, corn, and diced tomatoes. Bake until peppers are tender and serve with a side salad.
- **Lentil Soup**: Cook lentils with carrots, celery, onions, and garlic in vegetable broth. Season with thyme, bay leaves, and a touch of sea salt.
- **Spaghetti Squash with Marinara**: Roast spaghetti squash and top with homemade marinara sauce made from cherry tomatoes, garlic, basil, and olive oil.

Snack Ideas:

- **Trail Mix**: Mix raw almonds, walnuts, dried cranberries, and cacao nibs for a healthy, energy-boosting snack.
- **Fruit and Nut Bars**: Combine dates, almonds, and shredded coconut in a food processor. Press into a pan and refrigerate until firm, then cut into bars.
- **Herbal Tea**: Enjoy a soothing cup of burdock root or dandelion root tea.

Testimonials and Success Stories

Many individuals have experienced significant health improvements by following Dr. Sebi's alkaline diet and lifestyle. These testimonials and success stories illustrate the transformative power of his approach.

Testimonial 1: Reversing Chronic Illness

"I was diagnosed with type 2 diabetes and struggled with managing my blood sugar levels. After learning about Dr. Sebi's alkaline diet, I decided to give it a try. Within a few months, my blood sugar levels stabilized, and I lost weight. I no longer need medication, and my energy levels have never been higher." - Sarah, 45

Testimonial 2: Improved Digestive Health

"For years, I suffered from chronic digestive issues and bloating. Traditional treatments didn't help much. When I switched to Dr. Sebi's alkaline diet, I noticed a significant improvement in my digestion. I feel lighter, and the bloating is gone. I can't believe the difference it has made." - Mark, 38

Testimonial 3: Enhanced Vitality and Energy

"As a busy professional, I was constantly tired and relied on caffeine to get through the day. Dr. Sebi's diet changed my life. The plant-based, alkaline foods gave me sustained energy throughout the day. I no longer need coffee, and I feel more vibrant and alive than ever." - Jessica, 32

Testimonial 4: Skin Health Transformation

"I struggled with acne and eczema for years. Creams and medications provided temporary relief but never addressed the root cause. After adopting Dr. Sebi's diet, my skin cleared up, and I no longer have flare-ups. It's amazing how changing my diet improved my skin health." - Lisa, 27

Testimonial 5: Overall Well-Being

"I started Dr. Sebi's alkaline diet to improve my overall health. Not only did I lose weight, but I also noticed a significant improvement in my mood and mental clarity. I feel more balanced and in tune with my body. This lifestyle has truly transformed my life." - Michael, 50

These testimonials highlight the profound impact of Dr. Sebi's alkaline diet and lifestyle on individuals' health and well-being. By embracing his principles, many have found relief from chronic conditions, increased energy, improved digestion, and a greater sense of overall wellness.

Dr. Sebi's philosophy on alkalinization and health offers a holistic approach to wellness that emphasizes the importance of maintaining an alkaline internal environment. His diet, rich in natural, plant-based foods, along with his herbal remedies and practical lifestyle tips, provide a comprehensive framework for achieving optimal health. By understanding and implementing these principles, individuals can experience significant health benefits, prevent disease, and enhance their overall quality of life.

Embracing the Alkaline Lifestyle for Optimal Health

As we reach the end of this comprehensive guide, it's essential to reflect on the critical concepts we have explored and understand the profound impact an alkaline lifestyle can have on our health and well-being. Transitioning to an alkaline diet is not just about making dietary changes; it's about embracing a holistic approach to life that enhances our vitality, resilience, and overall wellness.

Understanding the Alkaline Diet

Throughout this book, we have delved into the foundational principles of an alkaline diet, inspired by the teachings of Dr. Sebi and other holistic health experts. At its core, the alkaline diet emphasizes consuming foods that help maintain the body's optimal pH balance. This balance is crucial for preventing diseases, reducing inflammation, and promoting overall health.

Key components of the alkaline diet include:

- **High Alkaline Foods**: Vegetables, fruits, nuts, seeds, and grains that contribute to an alkaline environment in the body.
- **Avoiding Acidic Foods**: Reducing intake of processed foods, sugars, dairy, and meats that lead to acidity and inflammation.
- **Hydration**: Drinking plenty of water, herbal teas, and natural juices to support detoxification and hydration.

The Role of Detoxification

Detoxification is an integral part of maintaining an alkaline lifestyle. Our bodies are constantly exposed to toxins from the environment, food, and stress. Regular detox practices help cleanse the body, support the liver and kidneys, and promote overall health. We have discussed various detox methods, including:

- **Liquid-Only Days**: Giving the digestive system a break by consuming only liquids for a day or two each week.
- **Salt and Soda Baths**: Using Epsom salts and baking soda baths to draw out toxins through the skin.
- **Low-Temperature Saunas**: Utilizing gentle heat to encourage sweating and detoxification.

Mental and Physical Practices

An alkaline lifestyle extends beyond diet to include mental and physical practices that reduce stress and enhance well-being. Integrating practices like walking, yoga, Tai Chi, and mindfulness can significantly impact your health. These activities:

- **Reduce Stress**: Lowering cortisol levels and preventing the body from becoming overly acidic.
- **Improve Circulation**: Enhancing oxygen delivery to tissues and organs.
- **Promote Relaxation**: Encouraging a state of calm that supports overall health.

Incorporating Dr. Sebi's Teachings

Dr. Sebi's insights into the relationship between alkalinity and health have provided valuable guidance for this book. His focus on natural, plant-based foods and the avoidance of processed and hybrid foods aligns perfectly with the alkaline diet principles. Key takeaways include:

- **Approved Foods**: Consuming foods from Dr. Sebi's recommended list, such as fresh fruits, vegetables, and whole grains.
- **Foods to Avoid**: Steering clear of foods that are highly acidic, processed, or contain artificial additives.

Practical Recipes for Daily Living

To make the transition to an alkaline lifestyle seamless, we have provided a variety of recipes that are both delicious and nutrient-dense. From breakfast options like Quinoa Breakfast Porridge and Avocado Toast to satisfying lunches like Chickpea Salad Wraps and Zucchini Noodles with Pesto, these recipes are designed to nourish your body while supporting your alkaline journey.

The Path Forward

Transitioning to an alkaline lifestyle is a journey that requires commitment, but the rewards are immense. By making conscious choices about what you eat, how you detox, and how you manage stress, you are investing in your long-term health. Remember that small, consistent changes can lead to significant improvements in your overall well-being.

Adopting an alkaline lifestyle is not just a dietary shift; it's a holistic approach to living that prioritizes health, vitality, and balance. Embrace the principles outlined in this book, experiment with the recipes, and incorporate the practices that resonate with you. Your journey towards optimal health and well-being begins now.

Appendix A: Testing Your First Morning Urine pH

Understanding Your pH Levels

Your first morning urine pH offers insight into your body's mineral reserve and its acid/alkaline state. The body uses overnight rest to excrete excess acids, and this capacity varies based on toxin load and individual abilities to generate energy, neutralize toxins, and excrete them.

How to Monitor Your pH

1. **Obtain Test Paper:** Get a packet of pH (HydrionTM) test paper with a test range of 5.5 to 8 from your local dispensary or pharmacist.
2. **Morning Test:** First thing in the morning, before urinating, cut off two or three inches of the paper tape.
3. **Wet the Tape:** Moisten the test tape with urine. For best results, ensure a 6-hour to 8-hour rest period before testing.
4. **Read the Results:** As the tape gets wet, it changes color, indicating the urine's acid or alkaline state. Compare the color of your strip with the chart on the back of the test tape packet and record your urine pH daily or as recommended by your physician.

Interpreting Your pH

- **Acidic or Alkaline:** A reading below 7.0 indicates acidic urine. The lower the number, the more acidic it is. Ideally, your first morning urine pH should be between 6.5 and 7.5. A neutral or slightly acidic pH suggests that your cellular environment is appropriately alkaline.
- **Low pH:** If your readings are below 6.5, you should consider dietary changes to alkalinize your diet. Initially, low pH readings are common due to the standard American diet's acid-forming nature. Occasionally, a reading between 7.5 and 8.0 is acceptable. Consistently higher readings indicate a "false alkalinity" and may suggest a catabolic state involving tissue breakdown.

Appendix B: Transit Time Digestion Evaluation

Purpose

Transit time measures the interval between consumption and elimination, indicating the efficiency of your digestive system.

How to Determine Transit Time

To evaluate transit time, we recommend using charcoal capsules, which are also used for symptomatic treatment of intestinal gas.

1. **Dosage:** Take 6-12 capsules (1.5-3 grams of charcoal) with 8 ounces of water between meals. Choose a high-quality.

   Dosage according to weight:

   < 150 lbs: 6 capsules

   150 – 200 lbs: 8 capsules

   200- 250 lbs: 10 capsules

   > 250 lbs: 12 capsules

2. **Timing:** For the most accurate results, ingest the capsules just after a bowel movement and note the time.
3. **Observation:** Monitor the consistency of your stool, noting changes in texture, color, and composition. Record the time when you first observe the black, crumbly, charcoal-like output.

Interpretation

- **Healthy Transit Time:** A transit time of 12-18 hours is considered healthy.
- **Long Transit Time:** Many Americans experience a transit time of 36-96 hours or longer. Prolonged transit times can lead to the absorption of digestive toxins and interfere with proper metabolism, increasing the risk of chronic illnesses.
- **Short Transit Time:** Very short transit times may not allow adequate digestion and assimilation of nutrients. Consult your physician or nutritional professional to determine the significance of your results and aim for a healthy transit time. It is recommended to recheck transit time twice a month until it normalizes.

Printed in Great Britain
by Amazon